CANCER:
A Coping Guide

for Those with the Big C

and Those who Love Them

Other published work from Elaine M. Decker

Retirement Sparks December 2011
Reigniting the Passion for Life—
Irreverent Observations on Retirement
Paperback
ISBN-13: 978-1468095708

New York Times

New Jersey Opinion: Sep 18, 1988
"Please Send One Bag of Garbage"
http://www.nytimes.com/1988/09/18/nyregion/new-jersey-opinion-please-send-one-bag-of-garbage.html

New Jersey Opinion: July 17, 1988
"Commuter Calls It Quits"
http://www.nytimes.com/1988/07/17/nyregion/new-jersey-opinion-commuter-calls-it-quits.html

Marketing News:

Viewpoint: May 11, 1992
"Being green is not as easy as it seems"

Viewpoint: April 15, 1991
"An open letter to Jim Manzi, Lotus president"

Privacy Journal

December 2000
"How to Track Missing Cats and Stray Husbands"

July 1990
"Assault with Intent to Sell"

CANCER:
A Coping Guide

for Those with the Big C

and Those who Love Them

by Elaine M. Decker

Published by Business Theatre Unlimited

Here's what those in the cancer field are saying about *CANCER: A Coping Guide:*

"In sharing her personal experience, Ms. Decker provides practical suggestions for... cancer patients, their families and friends to navigate this journey, adding her trademark satiric humor and leaving the reader in an upbeat mood."

-- Gary M. Calvino, Director of Development,
Gloria Gemma Breast Cancer Resource Foundation

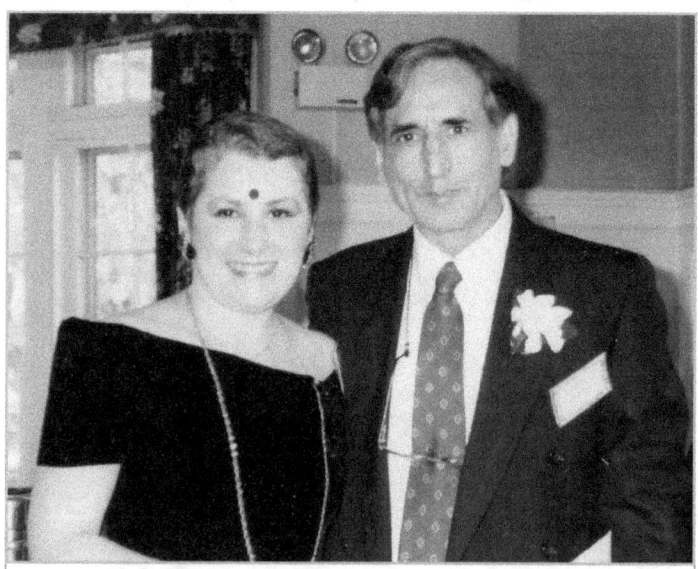

The author with her husband at their wedding reception in 1990, shortly after the completion of her treatment (chemo and radiation) for breast cancer.

Copyright 2012 by Business Theatre Unlimited
All rights reserved.
ISBN-13: 978-1479226511   ISBN-10: 1479226513

To Jagdish,
who found my tumor
and has been with me
throughout all the treatments
and the recovery
and
To Lyn and to Sheryl,
who fought the good fight
but lost the battle;
you are both still with me.

iv

Contents

Page

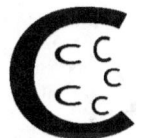

Contents (cont.)

Page

Introduction

I am a cancer survivor. I am also a writer. I'm known more for my humor and social satire, but I also write on serious topics. When I was diagnosed with breast cancer, I began keeping a journal of my own thoughts and experiences and those of others coping with many forms of cancer.

I wasn't quite sure what I would do with all the material I was collecting, but I assumed it would eventually find its way into a book. I am now a twenty-two year cancer survivor. That means *CANCER: A Coping Guide* has been twenty-two years in the making.

The book has three sections. The first, "Big C, Little cs," explores the range of emotions experienced by someone coping with cancer treatment. It also covers the difficulties with interpersonal relationships during this stressful time.

The second section, "Cancer Dos and Don'ts," is a guide to talking to someone fighting the disease. I've learned that many people have no idea what to say to a loved one with cancer. Equally importantly, they have no idea what *not* to say. You'll find ten dos and don'ts to help with this.

The final section is a humorous foray into what it means to be bald. "It's Good To Be Bald" is guaranteed to end your reading of *CANCER: A Coping Guide* with a smile.

My own battle began with a misdiagnosis. My doctor told me cavalierly and with great certainty, *"It's just a cyst. Come back in three months."* Then it was come back in six months, then eight.

His diagnosis was not based on a biopsy. He had simply looked at a six-month-old mammogram (done on antiquated equipment) that didn't seem to show anything where the lump was located.

Since the lump was growing and getting more painful, I eventually sought a second opinion. Though I lived in New Jersey, I traveled to Vermont to see a breast specialist recommended by my brother-in-law, who is an eye surgeon in that state. The specialist did a needle biopsy and within hours I had the bad news. I had stage two breast cancer.

The Lord works in strange ways, as common wisdom would say. That specialist was participating in a National Institutes of Health study of a new treatment protocol for breast cancer. I was randomized into the test cell and as a result, I had chemotherapy before my surgery.

At the time, this was not standard practice. It has since been shown to improve a woman's chances of long-term survival. I eventually learned that my tumor was composed of several fast growing, aggressive cancers. I also learned that the chemo had killed the cancer. (By the time I had my surgery, only the radioactive wire that had been inserted into the tumor before my chemo remained.)

In all likelihood, the test treatment saved my life. I wouldn't have received it from my initial doctor, because he was disinclined to use chemo and wasn't part of the NIH study.

This experience made me even more aware that once you have cancer, your treatment and your journey are ultimately in your own hands. Close friends and virtual strangers have similar stories to tell. We've discovered that knowing you are not the only one dealing with these issues can give you the courage and strength to move forward.

For years, I've been sharing the collective wisdom of my cancer circle with new people forced into our brotherhood. I've come to realize several things about coping with cancer. It is beyond frightening—it can be absolutely paralyzing. If it doesn't break you, it will probably make you stronger, but it could be years before you realize this.

As Americans' life expectancy increases, so, too, does the likelihood that more of us will experience some form of cancer during our lifetime. The inevitable result of this explosion is more and more people who have no idea how to interact with those of us battling the disease.

CANCER: A Coping Guide is for them, and through them, it is also for us.

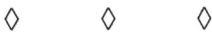

Section I

Big C, Little cs

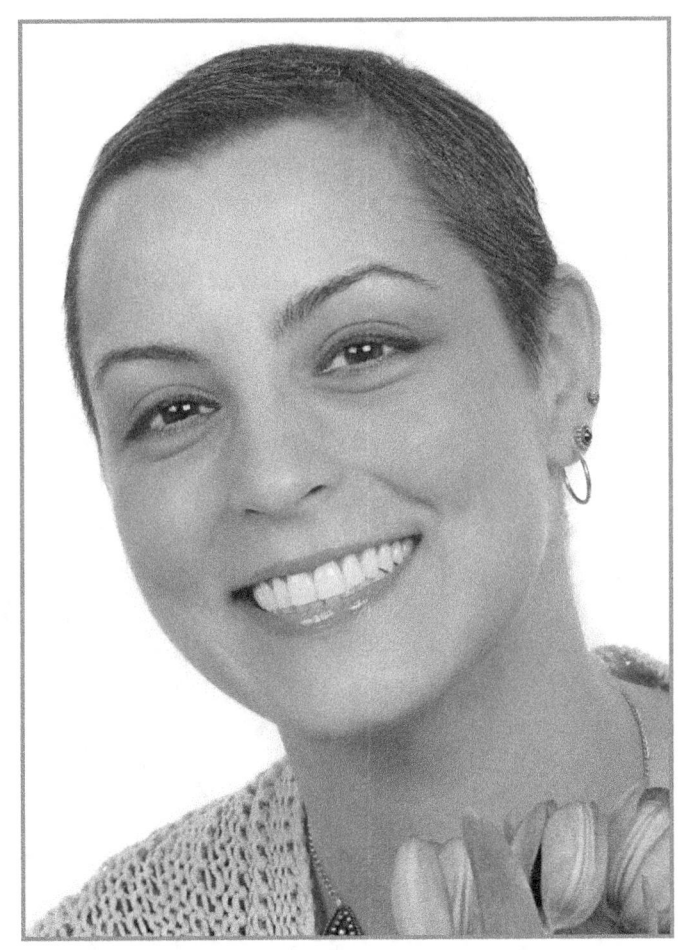

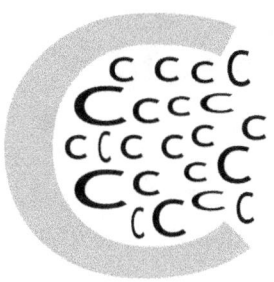

"The Big C" Brings Many Little cs Along with It

"The Big C." It's meant to be a euphemism, but it strikes almost as much fear in most of us as the word "cancer" itself. The phrase became a household word back when John Wayne, an American icon, made it known that he had developed the Big C.

As the population ages, more and more people are learning that they or someone they love has the Big C. It's become so familiar that one of the more celebrated TV shows is titled *The Big C.*

My father died of cancer many years ago. Sadly, several of my friends also succumbed to the disease. I'm fortunate to be a 22-year cancer survivor myself. Throughout my own treatment and my friends' over the years, I've learned that the Big C brings along with it many little cs.

Those little cs can have as much impact on a cancer patient's life as the disease itself, yet we're much less likely to hear about them. Patients who can manage the little cs will have a better chance of becoming a cancer survivor, like me.

Choices, Chances and Consequences

One of the first things a person with cancer learns about are the *choices* of treatments that are available and the *chances* of survival for each one.

Most of the choices are presented by a medical specialist and have a documented track record. Some of the choices come from well-meaning friends and loved ones, who often confuse you (another little c) more than help.

When you have cancer, the ultimate decision on which treatment you will undergo is yours and yours alone. You are the one who will live with the outcome of that decision and you should feel comfortable with it when you make it.

> *The decision on which treatment you will undergo ultimately is yours and yours alone.*

Evaluate your choices and chances. Consider the *consequences* of each one, including the side effects. Then go with the one that makes the most sense for you.

Sometimes those closest to you can be overbearing when they offer advice. Keep in mind that they're probably scared for you. They're just trying to help, often by researching every possible treatment.

When my husband learned I had breast cancer, he wanted me to consider a macrobiotic diet instead of the surgery and chemotherapy I had chosen. His friend's wife had beaten the Big C with macrobiotics after the medical community had given her 3 months to live.

I countered that for every person who did that successfully and hit the lecture circuit praising that approach, there are fifteen others who ended up in boxes in the ground and can't speak out against it.

After many tears and hurt feelings, we arrived at a compromise. I trusted my doctor and had more conventional therapy. But I also followed a low-fat diet with vitamin supplements, especially antioxidants, which

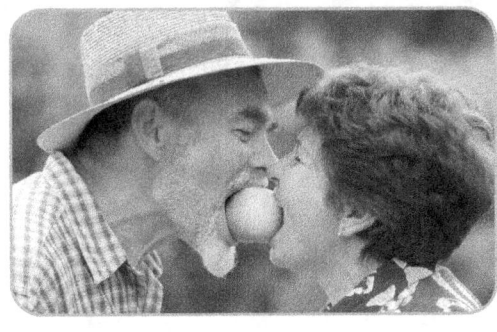 were not commonly accepted approaches back in the 1990's. I even took foul-tasting brewer's yeast, which gave a whole new meaning to the song *"What I did for Love."*

Each of the choices of treatments comes with its own chances of survival. Other than for knowing which treatment is relatively more successful than another, odds are often more destructive than constructive.

In the first place, they are nothing more than an accumulation of individual numbers based on individual cases. You can flip a coin twenty times and get twenty heads, and the odds are still 50-50 for it to come up heads again on the next flip.

If you are fortunate enough to have a cancer with high odds of survival, you can get complacent. If you have a particularly nasty type, you can get discouraged.

A close friend of mine, Lyn, had a rare and deadly type of bladder cancer. Her husband asked the odds question; (she didn't want to know). The 30% figure they were given seemed depressingly low to her.

I suggested another way to look at it. *"Suppose someone gave you a gun with six chambers and told you only two had bullets in them. Would you want to put the gun to your head and pull the trigger? I doubt it."*

That was about the same odds as the survival rate for her type of cancer. Suddenly, a 30% chance seemed pretty likely. Lyn and I agreed that the best way to keep our mental equilibrium was to forget the odds and concentrate on ourselves as individuals, doing everything we could to improve our own condition.

> *Forget the odds. Concentrate on yourself as an individual. Do everything you can to improve your health.*

For me, that included keeping my weight under control, eating healthier and getting regular exercise, even on days when I was tired and had to push myself to do it.

Today, there is far more information on diet and exercise and how that affects one's health. We also know how important getting enough sleep is to successfully fighting disease. And of course, reducing the stress level in our lives.

A few years ago, another dear friend found out she had stage four lung cancer. She had never smoked a day in her life; hers was another Dana Reeve's story. Not surprisingly, she was initially angry about the hand she'd been dealt. Her chances of survival were grim, and she wasn't certain she even wanted to undergo treatment.

Alexis was one of the smartest people I knew. We talked about the odds. *"All they are is a collection of data points,"* I reminded her. *"Someone has to be one of those outlying points—the exception, the success story. And it might as well be you. Behind the success percentages, no matter how low, are real people. People like you and me."*

Her fighting spirit kicked in and she opted for treatment. Though she eventually lost the battle, she had several months of improvement. That was several months spent with family and friends, all of us cherishing the time she had left.

My friend, Lyn, who had bladder cancer, participated in a research study that gave her more than a year beyond her expected time. During that year, she gambled in Atlantic City and attended a Neil Diamond concert at the NJ Meadowlands. Toward the end, she was able to see her son graduate from college. It was on video, not in person, but she lived to see it happen and to celebrate with him.

Mara was my college classmate, though I didn't know her well in school. When she was diagnosed with pancreatic cancer, one of the most deadly forms of the Big C, she started a blog where she eloquently chronicled her last months. Despite Mara's bleak prognosis, she chose to be grateful for every day she had left. She ended each post with *"Happy Thanksgiving!"* and she was an inspiration to us all.

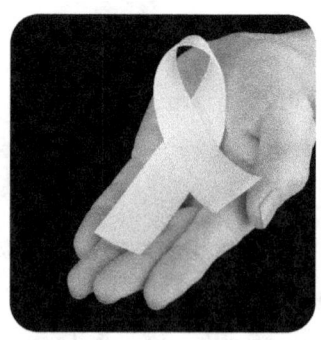

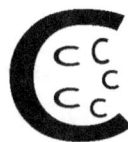

Contradictions—
Changes and Constants
Curiosity and Consideration

The Big C brings with it many *contradictions*. The most immediately noticeable is that everything around you seems to *change*, yet one thing will forever remain *constant*— *You have cancer*.

Your body changes. In many cases your hair falls out. You may get mouth sores and rashes. You are subject to nausea and diarrhea. You may go into instant menopause.

Your diet also changes. You'll probably be told to cut down on (or out altogether) caffeine and alcohol.

All these changes serve to remind you that you have cancer. For the rest of your life, no matter how many good checkups you will have, the threat and the fear of a recurrence will be hanging over you. It may get fainter over the years, but it will always be there.

The way people treat you changes, too, and more contradictions become apparent. For all the compassion (another c) people seem to have, a certain maudlin *curiosity* becomes apparent.

Mention that you are on chemotherapy and people immediately stare at your hairline to see if you're wearing a wig. Lyn warned me of this, and I contemplated getting a campaign-type pin that said *"Yes, it's a wig"* to put right up there where my part used to be.

Contrast this with the *consideration* shown by people who shave their own heads in support of family members and friends who have lost their hair during chemo.

Gary is the Director of Development for a regional breast cancer foundation. His job is to raise funds and increase awareness. He's an exceptionally compssionate person. At the foundation's headquarters, he shaved his own silver mane in solidarity with Donna, 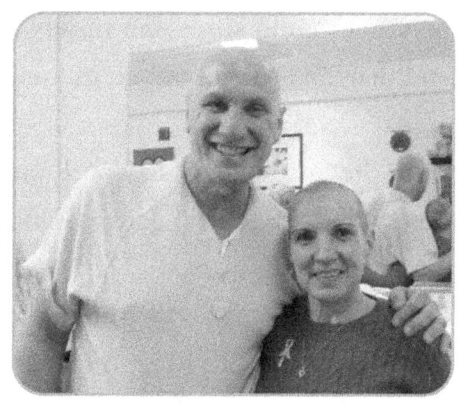 who was facing her second bout of chemo. This simple act of selflessness turned a solemn event into a joyous one.

There are so many moving stories about men and even children doing this to raise funds for cancer research and support services. Some organizations make the shave-a-thons an annual event. St. Baldrick's Foundation, in California, promotes them nationwide all year long.

Tell some people you were operated on for breast cancer, and they sneak sly looks from left to right, to see if one breast appears different from the other. Really inconsiderate "friends" start conversations on what the loss of a breast might do to the sexual relationship between husband and wife.

When you learn you have the Big C, you find out fairly quickly who your true friends are. They're the ones who are always considerate. They take their cues from you on what you're comfortable talking about. Be thankful for them and cherish them.

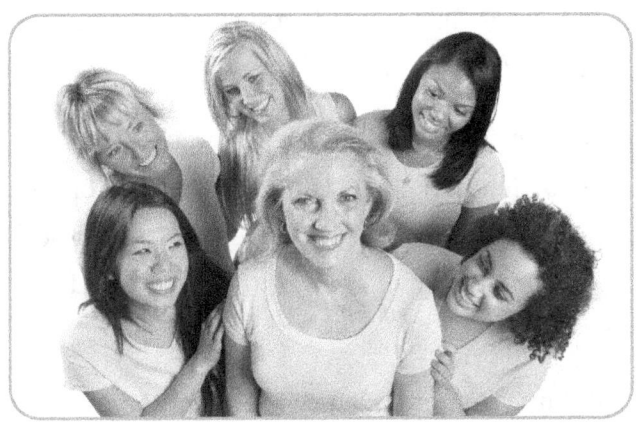

Forget about all the others.

No really. I mean it. Forget about them.

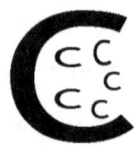

Control and Coping

One of the most difficult aspects of the Big C to deal with is the feeling of being out of *control*. You didn't ask for it and you can't just give it away. The more you can take back control, the better you'll be able to *cope* with the changes in your life.

The first way to take control is through your choice of treatment. Sometimes you don't like the choices before you, but it's important for you to be a party to the decision. It's one way for you to take control.

Make your decision and go with it wholeheartedly, whether it's chemo or macrobiotics, prayer or meditation. Think of yourself as in charge of what's happening to your body. You could have chosen any number of treatments, but you chose this one.

One of the most important ways to take control is to make sure you are facing in the right direction—forward and not backward. You can't change the past, and even if you could, it might not have made any difference.

Looking backward is negative energy; negative energy cannot beget positive results. Look toward the future, but don't try to plan too far out. Take each day as it comes, the first day of a future that you will control as much as you possibly can.

Lyn passed on advice that someone gave her: don't try to solve all your problems at once. Wake up in the morning grateful for the day that lies ahead of you and ask yourself what decisions need to be made, what problems overcome, to get through that day and that day alone.

That's good advice for dealing with any phase of life that has too many problems to handle with sanity. Take them one at a time, in the order that they hit you.

I found another way of coping that involves still another c— comparisons. By thinking of situations that would be worse, I made my own problem seem less burdensome. I could have had the bladder cancer that Lyn was fighting.

I could have been 34 years old with young children to worry about instead of 44 with none. I was able to direct all my energy into positive thinking. Had I been a mother, I would have had to at least consider the possibility that I might not survive, and to worry about who would raise my children.

I could have been healthy myself, but with a child who had leukemia. What mother with a child battling cancer would not try to make a deal with her God? *"Please give me breast cancer and let my child be healthy!"*

No matter how bad your cancer is, there must be some situation you can envision that would be worse. If there is just one person in this world with whom you would not want to trade places, you have a hook to help you cope and take control.

> *What mother of a child with leukemia wouldn't ask to have breast cancer in exchange for her child being cured?*

If you can't think of that one person in your own circle of family and friends, try watching a few hours of reality TV. You'll find dozens of programs that tell the stories of individuals and families that are undergoing hardships that are almost unimaginable. Some of those are sure to touch your own heart, leaving you feeling better off in comparison.

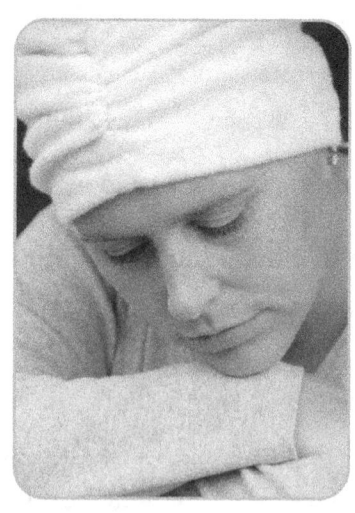

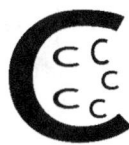 **Catharsis**

If you have anger about having cancer, it's important to express it, to get it out of your system. For some that involves crying or pounding fists; for others it involves talking the anger through rationally with someone.

> *If you're angry, get it out of your system; find a way to have your catharsis!*

For me, it involved transferring the general anger to one specific side effect of the treatment I had chosen. My second marriage took place in my forties, and—though it would have been a long shot—we hoped to have children. Chemo put me into premature menopause, so we would never be able to have a baby.

I wasn't so much angry at the cancer, but at the loss of the dream of a family. That was something more specific that I was able to cry about and then put behind me.

Whatever method works for you, experience your *catharsis* as soon as you can. Until you dispel the anger, you'll have difficulty coping and regaining control. But especially, you'll have difficulty keeping a positive attitude, which is key to fighting the Big C.

I tend to keep my deepest emotions to myself, or to share them with only my closest friends. When I discussed my cancer with most people, I was as rational as if I were talking about a lawn care service.

What surprised me was that the people I spoke with often got more emotional than I did. I finally realized that sometimes the people around you need to go through a catharsis, too. They may be fearful for you, or fearful for themselves, or irrationally guilty because they were spared and you got it.

Whatever the reason, they will cry into the phone and you will find yourself comforting them and assuring them that you'll be just fine. More often than not, this will happen only the first time they talk with you after they find out about your cancer.

If you know someone who persists in using you as a focus for their own catharsis, pass them on to someone else in your life to deal with. Otherwise, they'll drain your energy, and you need all of it to deal with the Big C—and all the little cs that come along with it.

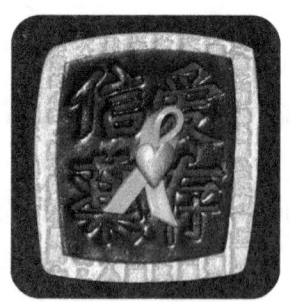

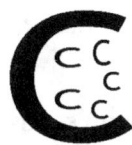 # Chuckles and Creativity

One of the best ways to deal with the stress of diagnosis and treatment is with humor. Research has shown that a positive attitude helps the immune system fight disease. Moreover, the ability to find humor in unlikely places can enhace your feeling of being in control.

Hard as it may seem, if you can *chuckle* about specific aspects of the situation, it will be easier to get through it. (Okay. I admit it. Chuckling is not the most elegant way to describe a sense of humor, but it's the only relevant word I could think of that starts with "c".)

One place to begin when looking for humor as a way to cope with cancer is to laugh at the side effects of the treatment. It helps to have a sense of humor when you're facing the prospect of waking up one morning to find your hair laying on your pillow and you've altready gotten out of bed. I penned "Ten Reasons It's Good to be Bald." You'll find it in Section III of this book.

People tend to take their cue from the patient when talking about any disease. If you're upbeat and positive, the people around you will be upbeat and positive.

The sisterhood of cancer sufferers shares an unusually strong appreciation for black humor. I was undergoing treatment at the same time as Lyn, my friend with bladder cancer. We went bald at the same time. We talked about putting on scads of makeup and oversized exotic earrings, and going to lunch in a fancy restaurant where no one would know us.

This was around the time that singer Sinéad O'Connor was popular, with her shaved head. The plan was to act as though we were models and bald was a cutting edge style. Sadly, Lyn's health never improved enough for us to realize our plan. But she never lost her sense of humor.

The more *creative* you can be in finding humor in your situation, the better. You'd be surprised at the ideas you can come up with, if you put your mind to it.

Chances are there's a local class on interesting ways to tie a scarf on your head. Enlist friends who like to cook in discovering recipes you'll enjoy while undergoing treatment. Ask your creative friends to plan fun, stress-free activities.

Surf the Internet for humorous photos of bald people. Challenge your support group to find the funniest photo. The winner gets to sign his or her name on everyone else's head.

Rent some comedy classics—The Three Stooges, Pink Panther movies, Austin Powers—and have marathon

CANCER: A Coping Guide

screenings with friends. Create a trivia quiz to go along with the movies you've chosen. (*"Oh! Behave!"*)

The possibilities are endless. Don't be shy about asking friends and family to bring chuckles and creativity to your life to help you cope with the Big C.

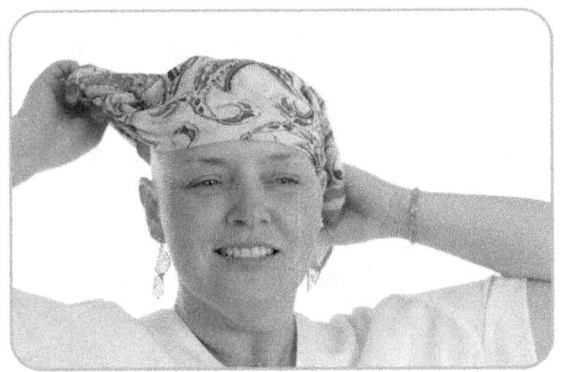

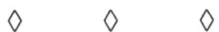

◊   ◊   ◊

CANCER: A Coping Guide

Section II

Cancer Dos and Don'ts

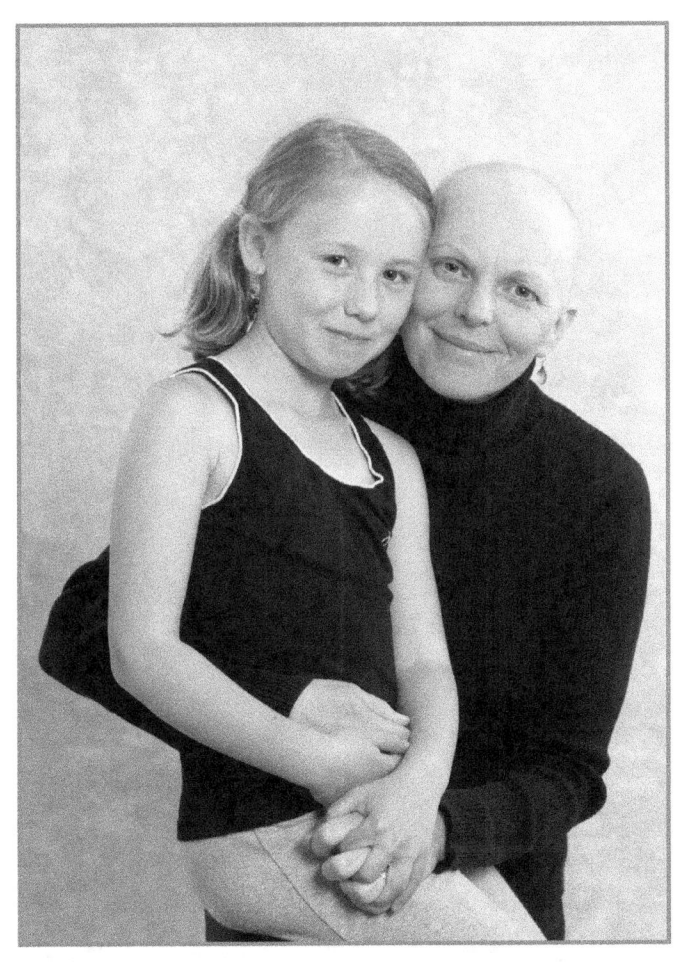

CANCER: A Coping Guide

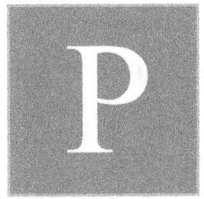 # Prologue

I am a cancer survivor. To the naked eye, I probably look a lot like you. Or your sister. Or your mother. But unless they are cancer survivors, too, we are not the same.

From a survivor's perspective, the world is divided into two groups: those who have personally battled the disease and those who have not. Survivors belong to a brotherhood they did not ask to join. But once they are members, they share an immediate bond with anyone forced into their ranks.

In the 22 years since I was diagnosed with breast cancer, I've lost many friends and relatives to cancer. Happily I've also celebrated many victories. I've also counseled dozens of family members, friends, colleagues, friends of colleagues and sometimes even strangers on ways to cope with this disease. We have cried together, laughed together, ranted, philosophized and cried some more.

My circle has included too many women with breast cancer, as well as men and women with skin cancer, prostate and uterine cancer, bladder and pancreatic cancer, colon cancer, brain tumors and lymphoma.

Our backgrounds are as diverse as our types of cancer and our reactions to the disease are as varied as our treatments. Over the years I've found a common thread within their stories: many of the people in their lives had no idea how to interact with them.

This was especially true during their initial diagnosis and treatment or toward the end of a battle it was clear they had lost—both times when they most needed understanding and support.

And it was true no matter what their relationship. Family members were just as likely to make missteps as casual acquaintances. Fellow cancer patients listening to these missteps typically nod knowingly, having had similar experiences of their own.

I've learned that if you have not had cancer yourself, you very likely are unsure how to approach friends, family and colleagues who have been diagnosed with this disease. A person with a deadly form—one for which there is no cure— is often treated like a pariah. Friends may go to extremes to avoid them, perhaps out of fear of catching the disease, irrational though that may be.

In the 1980's, I worked at a Fortune 500 company in New York City. We learned that one of our colleagues, a corporate attorney, was diagnosed with a rare and incurable cancer.

I remember seeing Jim eating in the cafeteria one day. Everyone else took a seat at another table, obviously avoiding him. He looked so alone that I went out of my way to sit with him. I could almost smell the fear that I saw in his eyes, but I could tell that he was grateful to no longer be alone, to no longer feel like a leper.

Every day thousands of people are diagnosed with some form of cancer. As a result, thousands of their family members and friends find themselves wondering what to say to them. Just as importantly, they're worried about what they should *not* say.

This section is for all of them, and through them, it's also for all of us.

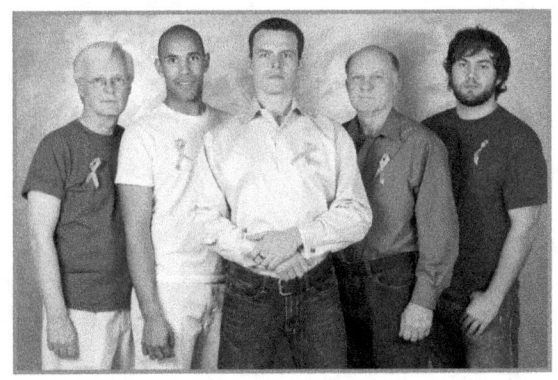

◊   ◊   ◊

CANCER: A Coping Guide

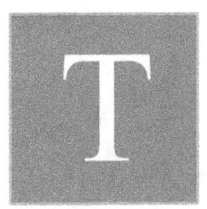 # Talking To Someone with Cancer

The latest statistics I've seen are that one in nine women is destined to have breast cancer (one in three, for women over age 60), and one in six men will develop prostate cancer. These are just two of many cancers that strike with little regard to age, income level or apparent health and fitness.

Eventually each of us will know someone who has cancer, which means each of us will face the question: What do you say to a friend, relative or co-worker who has it? Equally importantly, what *don't* you say to them?

People who have cancer have almost as many different ways of coping with the disease as there are types of cancer. One friend may openly share all the details of her treatment. Another might get offended if you ask any questions.

To further complicate your interaction, they often react differently from one day to the next. The first time you see them after their diagnosis, they may want to avoid the issue entirely. Two weeks later, they might be wondering why you seem to be walking on eggs when the word "cancer" comes up.

Be Prepared

Despite these differences, you can learn to be a supportive friend or loved one. Be prepared for a relationship that will be filled with contradictions, because that's what their life will have become. Some days even they won't be sure what mood they're in.

First and foremost, take your signals from the patient. If he doesn't seem to want to talk about it today, don't probe. Be prepared to talk about other things, things you would have discussed before you knew he had the disease.

When you do talk about it, don't be afraid to use the word "cancer." Euphemisms like "your illness" or "your problem" are like saying "your loss" or "his passing" instead of the word "death." We all know we must face death eventually, but fewer people expect to have to face cancer.

Avoiding the word makes most cancer patients feel what they have is too horrible to even mention. If you seem uncomfortable talking about it, your friend will feel more so. This can place a wall between you when he needs you most.

Keep in mind that everyone reacts differently. If your loved one clearly gets upset on hearing the word "cancer," back off until he can use it himself.

Be Sensitive

So what exactly should you say and what not? While there are no guaranteed rules, there are helpful guidelines. Many are just common sense, but it's amazing how often people fail to use it.

Cancer patients regularly hear well-intentioned, but nonetheless insensitive comments. Comments that appear innocuous, but can be painful to a person with cancer.

I lost my hair on chemotherapy. As soon as it started to grow in, I stopped wearing wigs and scarves, especially around family. One evening, my husband's 6-year-old niece looked at my bristly scalp and said: *"You look like a monkey."*

I imagine she was thinking of Curious George, but it took every ounce of my self-control to not start to cry. Because of the innocent source, I sucked it up. I can assure you that the same comment from an adult would have elicited a far more different reaction. *("Well, you look like a beached whale."* Or maybe, *"You smell like a wet cocker spaniel.")*

Situations like this will inevitably occur. If you know someone has cancer, think before you speak. If you make a misstep, don't take your loved one's reaction personally. If someone around you says something insensitive, help smooth things over.

My friend, Lyn, who participated in the bladder cancer research study, told me her oncologist warned her that the experimental drugs in the protocol were exceptionally potent and she'd be ultra-emotional during treatment.

This is how he described it to her. *"You'll feel as though your fingers and toes are ten feet long."* What an apt metaphor!

People can give someone undergoing treatment a wide berth. They can keep an emotional distance beyond what any reasonable person would expect. And they can still step on toes and hurt feelings.

Be assured that it's probably not you. It's the damn disease and the wretched treatment.

Listen

Keep in mind that often the best way to talk to someone with cancer is to *not* talk, but to simply listen.
Really listen.

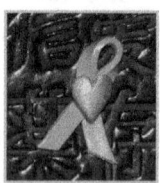

Give A Hug

Unless your friend or loved one seems totally averse to any physical contact, don't be afraid to touch them when you talk to them.

For someone coping with cancer, a hug can be worth a thousand words.

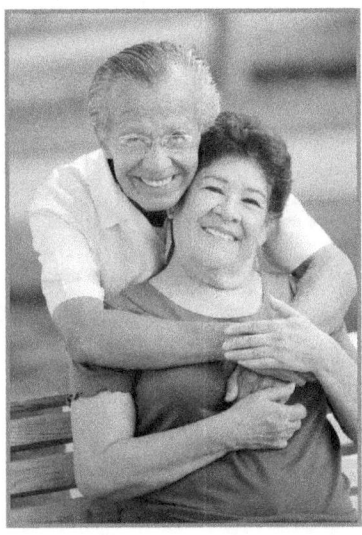

To help you interact with friends and loved ones coping with cancer, I've gathered ten things to avoid saying and ten to say freely.

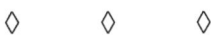

CANCER: A Coping Guide

10 Things *Not* To Say
To Someone with Cancer

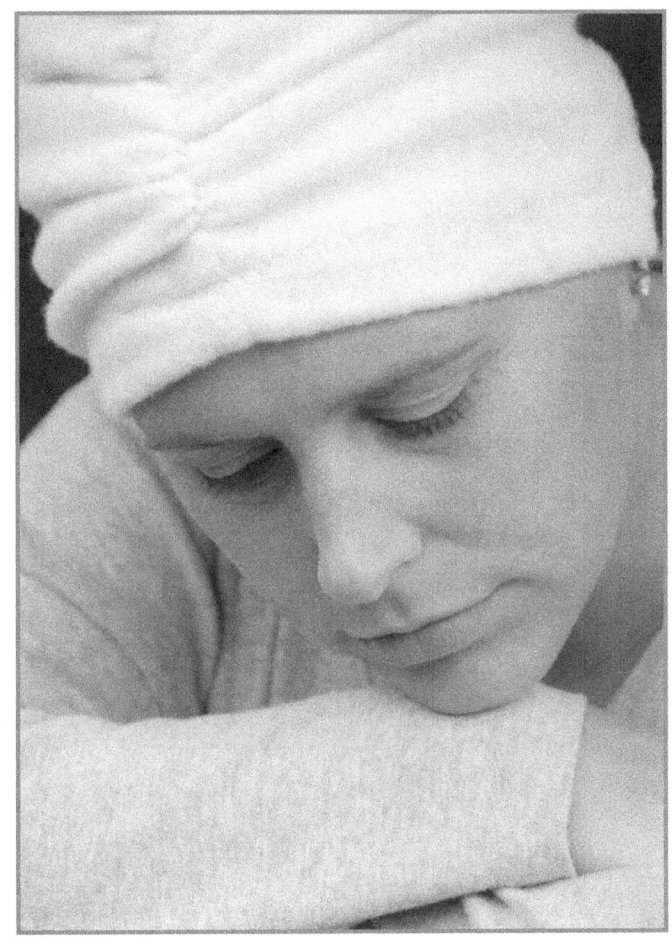

CANCER: A Coping Guide

1

They can do so much for cancer these days.

This is one of the most common things a person with cancer hears.

It can be appropriate if it's reinforcing what your friend has expressed to you. It should not be the first thing you say when you hear about the cancer.

Yes, it's true that the medical profession has many weapons in the modern arsenal against this disease.

But it's still hell to have it; and no matter how many good check ups he will ever have, he'll never be sure it's gone.

If your friend provides details on his planned treatment, be supportive. *"That sounds encouraging"* is a comment that is safe. It's not likely to draw you into a discussion that he should be having with his doctor instead.

If you find yourself unable to avoid a conversation on what "they" can do for cancer, be sure to frame it in the proper context.

If you're a cancer survivor yourself, say *"Here's what I found when I was a patient."* If you've gained insight from another friend battling the disease, say *"This is what one of my other friends told me about his treatment."*

Never phrase things as expectations for your loved one's outcome.

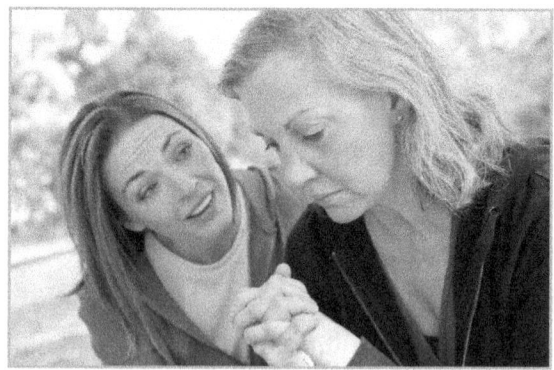

2

Everything's going to be okay.

Everything is *not* going to be "okay."

For the rest of her life, she will live with the threat and very real fear of a recurrence.

While you don't want to project or reinforce a feeling of gloom and doom, a perky Polyanna attitude can be equally inappropriate. It makes it appear that you don't appreciate the seriousness of the problem.

It's great to encourage a positive mindset, but do that by saying *"You're going to get through this. I'll help you."*

Be sure to ask *how* you can help.
"What can I do to make this journey less difficult for you?"

Notice I did not say "easier." For most cancer patients, it will not be easy, so "easier" is not an option.

Do be sure to talk in terms that indicate you expect your loved one to be around for a long time.

If he's reached the stage in his disease where you both know that's not the case, talk instead about events in the near future that you can hope to share.

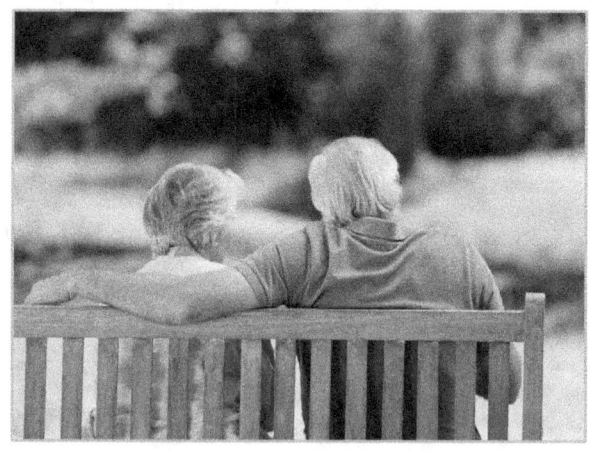

3

You look so healthy! I can't believe you have cancer.

Although this is meant as a compliment, it can have a negative impact.

A person with cancer is more sensitive than usual and may perceive this as questioning the truth or seriousness of his situation. Moreover, he has probably been struggling with his own denial phase.

Hearing someone else affirm that he doesn't look sick makes it that much more difficult to face the fact that he is.

(Compare this to item eight under what you *should* say.)

Compliment him on his tie, his shirt, his shoes.

If it's a woman, it's best to avoid hair and makeup, unless she seems to be fishing for a compliment.

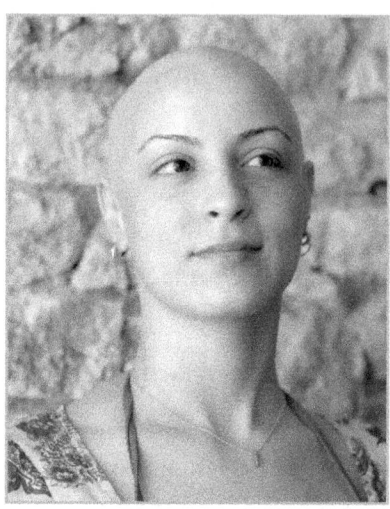

Even then, be careful. Her hair and her complexion are some of the first places where the side effects of her treatment will begin to show up. She may be worrying that others will notice it.

"That style is very becoming" is much safer than *"I've never seen your hair looking better."* (See also item six.)

4

So-and-so has a cousin who had your type of cancer, and she said...

One of the hardest struggles a cancer patient has is maintaining her individuality instead of becoming just another statistic.

Everyone is different and reacts differently to treatment. Third-hand information is usually wrong or misleading anyway. (Remember the childhood game of telephone...)

Worse, this comment sets up a comparison on behavior, coping, and expected results.

It's much better to offer this connection as a network for support, saying *"I know someone who recently had a similar diagnosis. You might find it helpful to talk with her."*

If your friend seems receptive to this, offer to make the initial contact and introduction.

Be sure to emphasize the fact that everyone's situation is different. Encourage your friend to speak with several others with her type of cancer. It will give her an idea of the range of experiences she may encounter.

Follow up to see if she's reached out to others. Don't nag; rather, gently encourage.

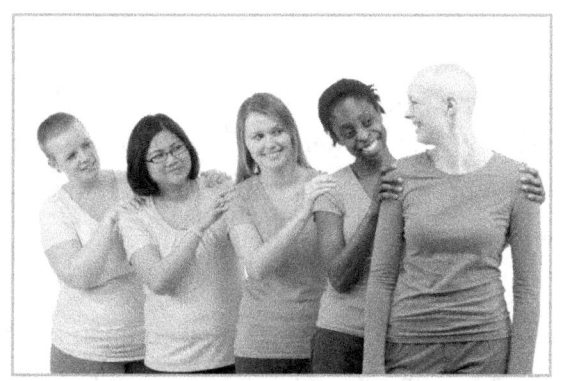

$$5$$

Do you need the name of a good doctor?
Or: Have you considered alternative therapy?

A key link to a cancer patient's recovery is trust in his doctors and hence the treatment they recommend. Such questions only lay the groundwork for second-guessing them.

If your friend appears to lack trust in his doctors, by all means encourage and help him to seek more information or a second opinion. Don't plant the seed of doubt through your own questions.

If you have good reason to believe his doctor is not qualified to handle his treatment, you can suggest questions he might want to ask or research that might be useful for his treatment. You should not bring this up in your first conversation after his diagnosis.

For more than eight months, my own tumor was misdiagnosed as a fibrous cyst. I eventually sought a second opinion in another state, where my physician brother-in-law could recommend a specialist I would trust. I chose to have my initial treatment and surgery there, as well, since I could recuperate with my sister.

Some months later, I discovered that one of my former co-workers was also undergoing treatment for breast cancer. Her doctor was the one who had misdiagnosed me.

I never told her that. She was well along in her treatment at that point and not likely to change horses mid-stream.

Sharing my own story would only have sown seeds of doubt for her. It would not have been constructive. I knew that having confidence in her doctor and her treatment was important to having a successful outcome.

Today, she, too, is a twenty-two year cancer survivor.

Your wig looks terrific!

This is another comment that is meant as a compliment but can backfire because of your loved one's magnified sensitivity.

It can come across as criticism of the way her own hair looked. Besides, the wig is hot and it itches and it has been forced on her, no matter how good it looks.

"Is that your hair?" is equally insensitive and morbidly curious.

If asked, say something positive (*"That style looks great on you"*), but don't volunteer your opinions.

Be especially careful of what you say if you're not absolutely certain it's a wig. If your friend hasn't specifically acknowledged she's wearing one, she may think it's so natural looking that most folks won't notice. Indeed, that's often the case with today's wigs. (Unlike twenty-two years ago!)

Even if you think hers is obviously a wig, don't burst her bubble. There will be plenty of other people around to do that.

When I was undergoing treatment for my breast cancer, I was working as a consultant three days a week. The Executive Director knew about my situation, but the staff did not.

Since I expected to go bald, I told people I was considering cutting my hair and biting the bullet and finally coloring my gray.

The first time I wore my wig, several people told me how much they loved my new hairstyle. A few of those who had known me for quite awhile confided: *"You should have dyed your hair years ago! It looks so much better."*

On several occasions, I came within an inch of yanking the wig off my head and shouting, *"I'm bald, damn it."* Not a pretty picture.

7

You're lucky you have such a strong marriage. Your husband won't care if you have your breast removed.

(Or: if you lose your sex drive.

Or anything else that raises the prospect of the problems your friend may have to face as a result of the cancer or its treatment.)

No matter how well-intentioned, this is the wrong thing to say.

You don't know what goes on behind closed doors in someone else's home. The marriage may not be as strong as you think and even the strongest are strained by dealing with cancer.

Your friend doesn't want to be reminded that more adjustments may lie ahead. The fear of changes in close relationships is one of the more difficult emotional aspects of coping with cancer, no matter how secure someone felt before.

Encourage your friend to gather a network of supportive friends and family around her. Make sure your name is at the top of the list of those she can call when she feels she needs to talk.

Find information on local support groups for others facing the same challenges.

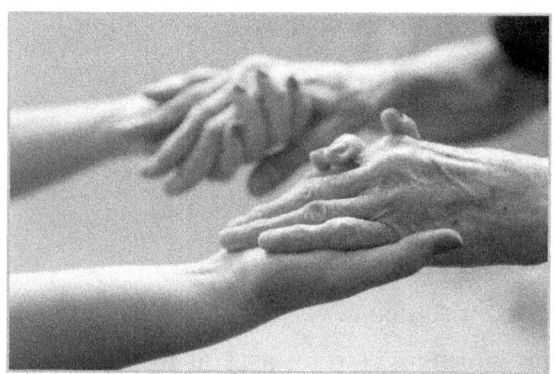

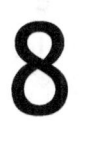

How are your children handling it?

The cancer patient probably isn't sure himself how his children are handling it. Children often deny the cancer even more than patients do. They believe we are all indestructible and immortal.

Your friend probably has a lot of guilt over the disruption this is causing in his family. He may also have fear over who will care for them should the worst happen.

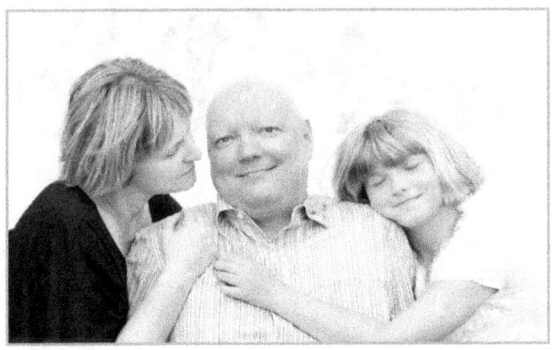

It's okay to ask if you can help with them in anyway. Can you give them rides to sporting events or dance recitals? Have them over to your house for a pizza party?

If your loved one brings up the subject of her children herself, offer to research some books that can help with this. There are a number of excellent ones available as any on-line search will show.

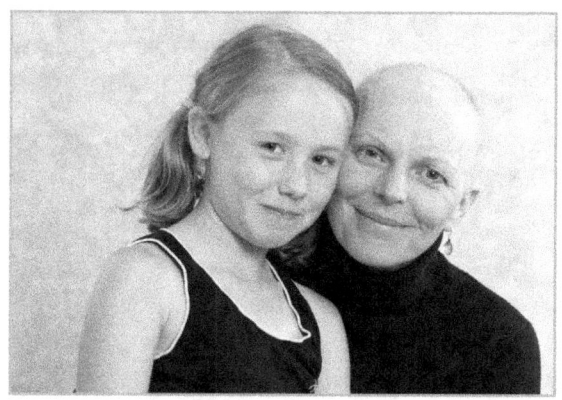

9

No one said it would be easy.

(Or the opposite approach: I feel so sorry for you.)

Indeed, no one did, and it isn't.

You shouldn't encourage a cancer patient to feel sorry for herself or to complain constantly. There's ample data that having a positive attitude is one of the best tools a cancer patient can have in his arsenal. But it's not always easy to be cheerful when you feel rotten.

If your friend complains, it's okay to show understanding, but avoid excessive sympathy. Try *"I'm sure it's not easy; is there anything I can do to help?"* instead.

If your loved one is in the final stages of the battle and there truly is no hope left, it's still important to help him avoid self-pity.

Whatever days he has left will be richer if he can focus on whatever joy is left in his life— and everyone has some joy, if he looks hard enough.

There are tactful ways to turn the conversation to a more upbeat, constructive note. Avoid the usual controversial topics of politics and religion, even if those used to be okay.

Suggest going through photo albums of shared memories. Was there a foolish joint excursion in your past that always makes you laugh when you recount it?

All of us have some of these stories that never lose their luster in the retelling. Scour your own memory for a handful of them as your go-to tools to change the tone of the conversation.

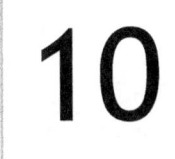

I would have called you sooner, but I didn't know what to say.

This is the lamest excuse, but sadly, one of the most common.

It can make the cancer patient feel guilty for burdening you with figuring out what to say. It frames her as a cause of stress in your life.

It can also make her feel you place a low priority on her friendship.

You didn't care enough to really try to come up with something to talk about.

You didn't value her enough to put yourself in an uncomfortable position, to be inconvenienced.

It makes her feel abandoned and alone at the one time when she most needs the support of

people who were an important part of her life
before she was diagnosed.

Someone who really cares can always think
of something to say.

If you honestly can't, relax.
And read on.

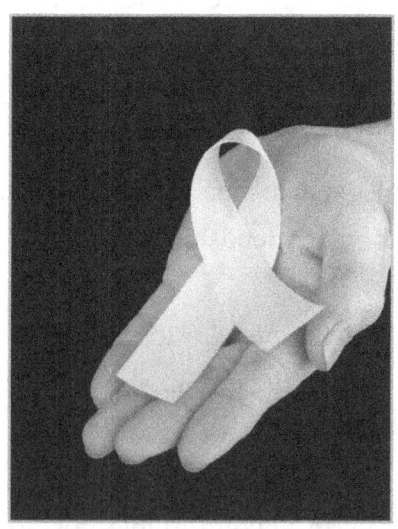

10 Things You *Should* Say
To Someone with Cancer

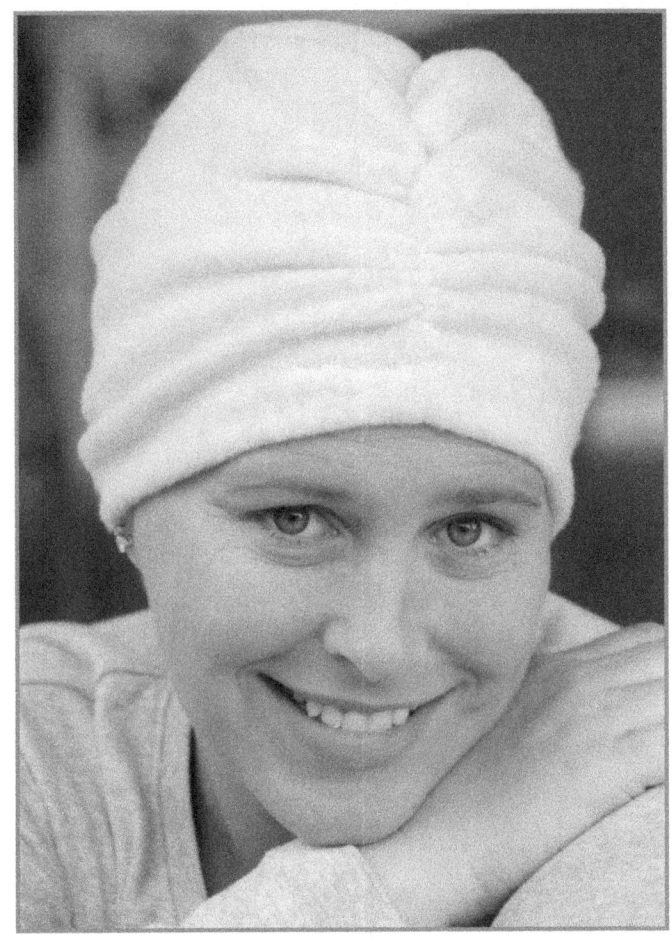

CANCER: A Coping Guide

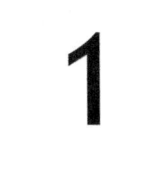

Do you want to talk about it?

This lets the cancer patient set the framework for your conversation. If he says "no," respect this and move on to other topics that you might normally discuss.

If he says "yes," follow with, *"Is there any aspect of your cancer that you don't want to talk about?"*

Let him take the lead on what to discuss, being careful to avoid anything he says is off-limits.

Whatever he chooses to talk about, remember to be a good listener.

Pay attention to even the littlest details. If he circles back to them later and you don't remember what he said, you'll seem insincere.

Be prepared for him to be repetitive to the point of obsession. For many cancer patients, that's their way of working out the things that are still unclear.

Don't be afraid to repeat back to him some of what he is saying to you. It shows you're truly listening. Just be careful not to parrot his exact words, or he may feel you're being patronizing.

Sometimes, just hearing his thoughts spoken out loud helps a patient in the decision-making process. Hearing his ideas played back to him can validate them.

It can also help him to avoid poor choices or to realize that some of them haven't been fully thought out yet.

If you think about it, this is true for most decisions, health or otherwise. It's especially true when it comes to facing the Big C.

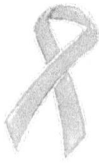

2

This must be awfully difficult to deal with.

This helps the cancer patient who wants to talk, but has trouble beginning. It opens the door for her to talk about what, specifically she finds difficult to deal with.

It shows understanding without encouraging self-pity. It gives her permission to admit she is scared or worried and it opens the door to framing possible next steps in a positive way.

One of the things I always recommend for those dealing with cancer—their own or a loved one's—is to practice what I call "emotional triage."

Take one day at a time and don't try to look too far out. Deal with the most important and immediate issues first.

Ask: *"What do we have to decide today?"* For anything else on the list, say: *"Let's worry about that when the time comes."*

Giving a patient permission to defer worrying about at least a few of the issues on her plate can be a gift beyond measure.

It can help her focus on the important decisions that need immediate attention. It can reduce the stress she is feeling.

All of this can lead to better decisions, and that usually means better outcomes.

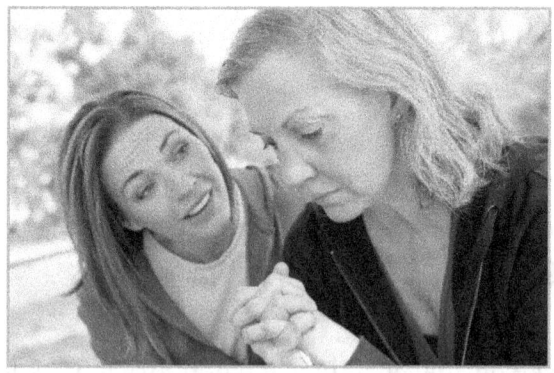

3

I just called to see how you're doing today.

This is just as simple and direct as it sounds.

If things are going well, show that you're happy for your loved one.

If they are not going well, listen with patience and understanding. After an appropriate interval, look for ways to brighten the conversation or redirect it.

Talk about trips you've taken together or family gatherings.

Find out if he's reading any books that he would recommend. Then borrow one from him so you can talk about it the next time you call. Have in mind some books that you've read that you think he'll enjoy.

Tell him that you've been appointed the official contact person from his circle of friends to check in and report on how things are going.

Ask if he has any particular message he'd like you to bring back to them. Jokingly suggest that if you go back empty handed you'll be in big trouble.

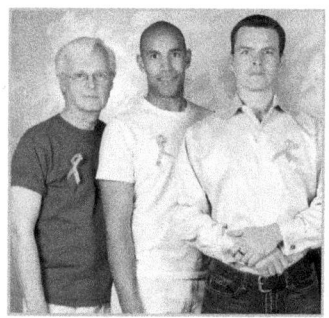

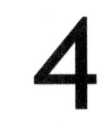

I admire how well you're handling this.

Or: I think it's terrific that you're putting one foot in front of the other and doing what you have to do.

This is important to say even if he isn't handling it that well. It encourages him to live up to the compliment and have the courage to do what must be done.

Most cancer patients would like to be brave about what they're facing, but it isn't always easy to do.

If you've learned that they've cut back on caffeine, be sure to give them kudos for that. Tell them you know how hard it is to give up that second (or third) cup of coffee.

Remember that what may seem like simple accomplishments to someone healthy can be Herculean to someone fighting cancer. This is especially true when they are on chemotherapy or undergoing radiation.

Go out of your way to uncover those simple things and genuinely praise them.

Think about your own (hopefully) normal life. Are you always brave? How easy is it for you to be brave? What's the scariest situation you can remember facing?

Multiply this ten times and you still won't have any idea how difficult it is for someone facing the Big C to be brave.

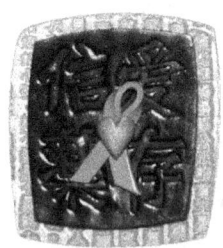

5

You don't owe anybody any explanations for anything.

Or: You're entitled.

Dealing with cancer frazzles the emotions.

Chemotherapy often makes people ultra-sensitive. Your loved one may get angry over something trivial or may cry over what seems to be nothing.

Afterward, she may feel guilty about what happened. She shouldn't blame herself for behavior that is to a large extent out of her control.

It's particularly important to reassure her if she is recounting something that happened with a person who was less understanding. Or perhaps didn't know about the cancer.

I was undergoing chemotherapy when I was engaged, but few people knew. It was highly likely the chemo would put me into premature menopause.

My fiancé and I were at a party where I met some people for the first time. A friend of his niece asked if we were planning to have children and I burst into tears. She was confused and felt terrible that such a simple question would upset me.

She didn't know that I had cancer. And she certainly didn't know that I was on chemo and it was slamming the door on any chance of having a family with my soon-to-be husband.

I felt bad that I had upset her. Then I had to explain why her question made me cry, which made things even worse for me.

I wish someone there had known to say to me: *"Don't feel bad that you cried. You're entitled."*

6

I've been thinking about you.

And (if both you and the person with cancer are religious):
I've been praying for you.

Many times a person with cancer drops out of sight while he's undergoing treatment. It can boost his morale (and his ego) to know that he hasn't been forgotten.

That you've been thinking about him reinforces his value as a person. It makes him feel he's still part of his regular world, even if he's not being seen in it.

If he is not religious, be careful about mentioning your prayers. It may make him uncomfortable and he may feel you think he's dying. Talk instead about recollecting something you've done together, an interest you share, and your hope to do it again soon. Plan ahead for this type of conversation.

Picture your loved one and what first comes to mind when you think of him. Is it his smile? His walk? A particular jacket he wears? An ugly old hat?

Tell him you saw someone with that same smile or walk, or a similar jacket or equally ugly hat, and it reminded you of him. This is one time when a little white lie can be a good thing.

Reflecting on something that may seem trivial to you can bring a rare and welcome sense of normalcy to a cancer patient's life.

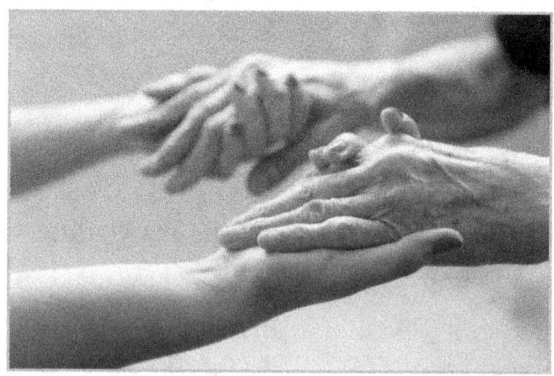

7

Would you like to have lunch (dinner) next week?

Or: Let's go shopping; bring your credit cards!

Or: Let's go down to Murphy's Sports Bar and catch the Red Sox (Yankees, Knicks, Lakers, Pats, Jets) game.

This adds some normalcy to the cancer patient's life and the best thing you can give him is your time.

To the extent he is physically able, he should continue to do the things he did before he had cancer, but he may be reluctant to initiate them. Be prepared to make adjustments. If you go fishing, he may have to do it from a chair on the beach and for just an hour or two.

Keep in mind that your friend's treatment may prevent him from drinking alcohol. If you go to a bar and he has to pass on the alcohol, order something non-alcoholic, too.

Joke that you've always been curious about Near-Beer. Tell him: *"I know you'll do the same for me if I ever need it!"* This reinforces the fact that cancer can happen to anyone and it's not your friend's fault.

Keep the ground rules the same. If you always went "Dutch," don't try to pick up the tab. This may draw attention to his medical bills, which could be a source of stress.

If you know finances are a real problem, ask *"Can I pick this up this time?"* This implies there will be a next time and that maybe he'll pick it up then. Don't make him think you feel sorry for him, or worse—that you think he has only a few more lunches left in his life.

If your loved one is nearing the end of his battle, it's even more important to bring some semblance of normalcy to what time he has left. You might have to adapt your usual routine to his limitations.

Suggest a quiet card game or even just sitting and reading together. Offer to read out loud from a book you know he'll enjoy.

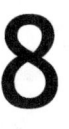

I hope you feel as good as you look today.

This is one the best things you can say to a cancer patient if it is even reasonably appropriate.

Many people with cancer look healthy throughout most of their treatment. It can make your friend feel better to know he doesn't look as though he's at death's door.

Obviously, this is not something to say when he truly looks awful. (Note the difference between this comment and the third one under the "Don'ts.")

If he is not looking particularly well, see if there's any aspect of his appearance that looks reasonably good and comment on that.

Perhaps he's walking a bit faster. *"It seems like you have more energy today. I hope you feel that way."*

Maybe there's something about her that seems improved from the last time you saw her. Tell her: *"Your color looks better this week. I hope that's a good sign."*

Note the difference between this—color—and complexion, which is better to avoid. (See item five under "Don'ts.")

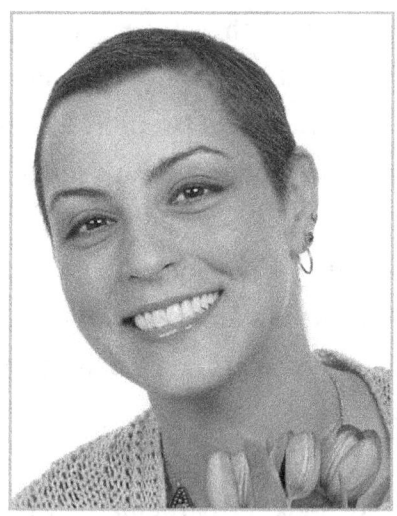

If your loved one has been looking and feeling marginal, this can lift her spirits almost as much as a new pair of shoes will.

I'm here if you need me. Just call.

This is another one that's as simple and direct as it sounds. Be sure you intend to deliver if she calls.

Broken promises are disappointing to everyone; to someone with cancer they can be devastating. If you tell your friend that you'll help her get through it, be sure you mean it.

She may not have the energy to contact you on her own. Don't leave the monkey on her back. Tell her that if you don't hear from her in a few weeks, you'll call her. And do it.

Use the calendar on your computer or some other reliable tool to remind you when it's time to call again. We all get busy; you're only human. Find ways to make it easier for you to be a good friend when she needs you most.

Ask if you can stop by to check in on her from time to time. Tell her that it will make *you* feel better, but that you don't want to be a pest.

Remember, for most cancer patients, it's better to be pestered than ignored.

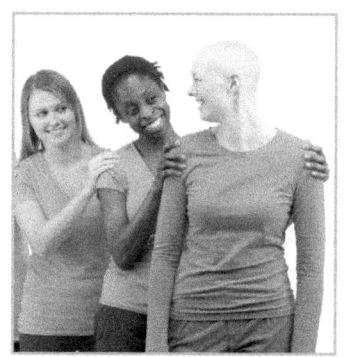

CANCER: A Coping Guide

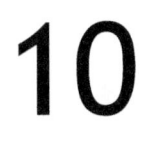

I love you.

Or: (If you don't sincerely feel that strongly) I care about you.

The most important thing you can communicate to someone with cancer is that you sincerely care about him and his problems.

Say it directly.
Say it with feeling.
And say it often.

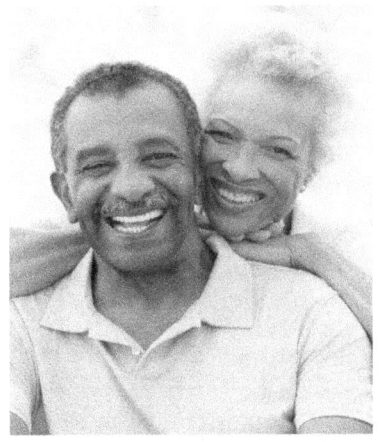

CANCER: A Coping Guide

Section III

It's Good To Be Bald

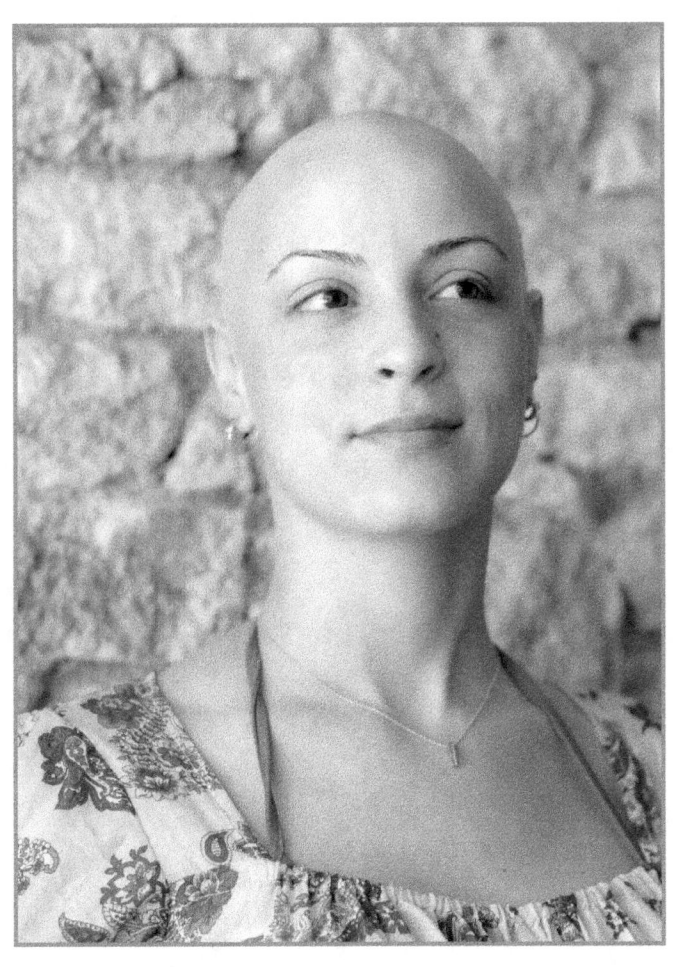

CANCER: A Coping Guide

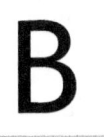 **Being Bald**

I lost all my hair when I was on chemotherapy. I got some wigs, but I hated how they felt. More often than not, when I went out, I tied a scarf on my head. (I learned that cotton or rayon were best; silk and polyester slipped around too much.)

As it turned out, I had a pretty nicely-shaped head underneath my hair. Or so I thought. Once, when I visited my mother and had my head covered with a scarf, I could tell that she was curious to see what my bald head looked like underneath. I told her I'd show her, if she promised not to cry when she saw it. She said she wouldn't.

As soon as I took off the scarf, her mouth started to crinkle up. *"Here come the waterworks,"* I thought. But instead, she burst into a fit of uncontrollable laughter. So much for my cute bald head.

My mother's laughter made me realize that the best way to deal with being bald was with a sense of humor. Since I'm especially known for my black humor, I wrote two pieces related to baldness: first, with a (bald) head nod to David Letterman, "10 Reasons It's Good To Be Bald," and second,

"The Great Hairs of History." I also drew some humorous sketches which I've used to illustrate Good To Be Bald.

"The Great Hairs of History" was a direct mail offer that I sent to friends and family. For $29.95, they received a lock of hair from some notable person, thanks to the wonders of cloning. In an effort to cheer me about my own baldness, my sister actually placed an order (under the *nom de plume* Ima Gotta Nohair). The order form for The Great Hairs, Ms. Nohair's letter and my company's response to her are at the end of this section.

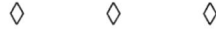

10

Reasons It's Good To Be Bald
(Unisex Version)

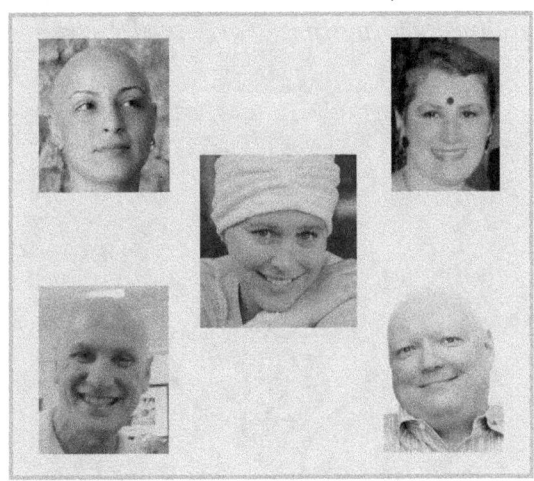

After your shower, you can blow-dry in a breeze.

No power? No problem! Just AIR dry.

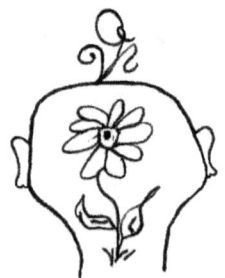

Environmental
beautification model

2

Your mother will finally stop telling you how to wear your hair (or for guys, to cut your hair).

Why must you always have it hanging in your eyes?

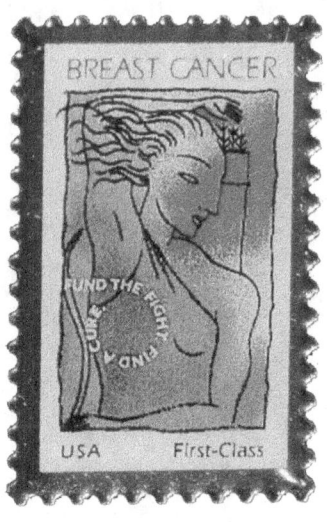

3

You'll save money on hair products, haircuts and stylings. (And you'll be done with the stress of the haircare aisle.)

Do I want the shampoo and conditioner combo? Or separate products?

Should I get the one for colored hair? Or the one for oily hair?

Is it gel or mousse that's "in" for metrosexuals this month?

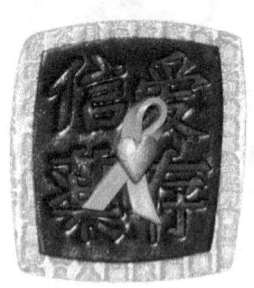

4

You've got the ideal place for that exotic tattoo you've always wanted.

No, it's not a red-footed booby. It's a lorikeet!

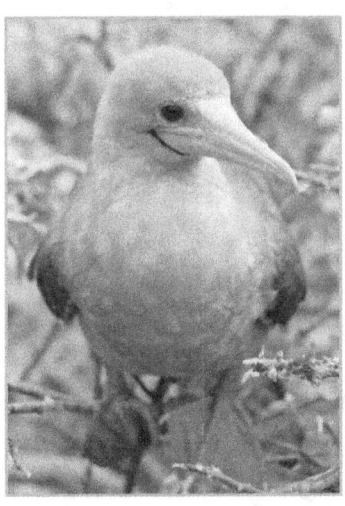

5

Your worries about dandruff are over.

Now you can focus on the cat hair...

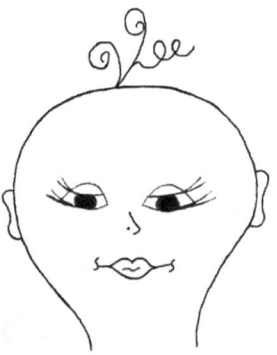

What do I care? Linda Goodman says
a Virgo's best feature
is her eyes anyway!

6

You can rent your head for local advertising.

Your Ad Here!

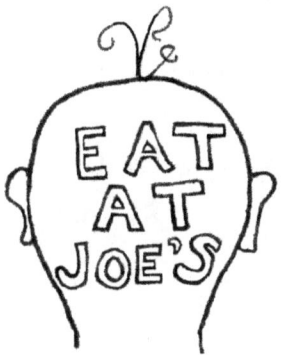

Revenue
generating
model

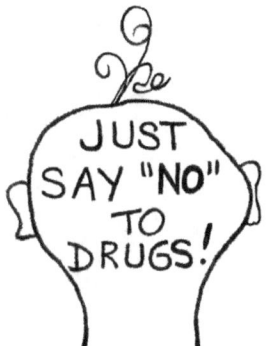

Public
sevice
model

7

There are no more stray hairs on the bathroom rug to get tangled around your toes in the morning.

But you still have to watch out for fur balls...

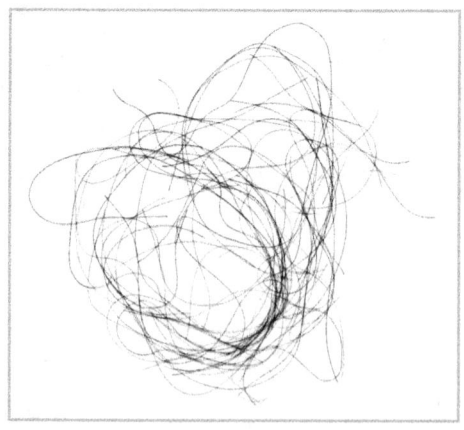

CANCER: A Coping Guide

8

Some of the best-loved figures in history were bald, including Gandhi, Churchill, and the Pillsbury Dough Boy.

Don't forget Kojak. And Yul Brynner.
How about Yoda? Plus James Carville and
Samuel L. Jackson. I could go on forever.

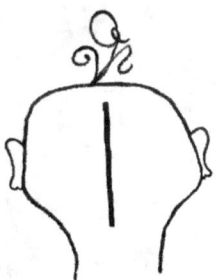

Headline. Or fine line. Or nohairline
I could still go on forever.

9

When you're lying in bed, it's much easier to tell where your head ends and the cat (or dog) begins.

Which is probably useless information in most pet homes.

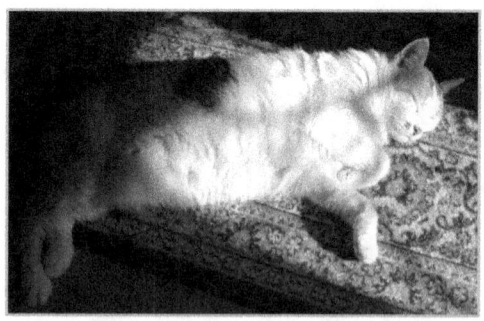

10

You can find out once and for all if your ears really are off-center.

You see, officer? I'm not tipsy! My ears are just crooked...

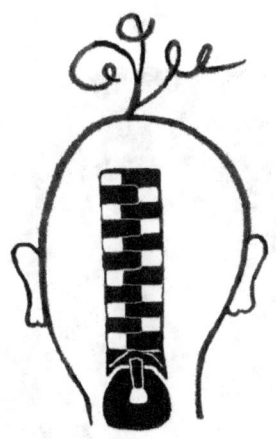

Trompe l'oeil model

3 BONUS Reasons for Women

You don't have to shave your legs and underarms anymore.

You don't have to touch up your roots anymore.

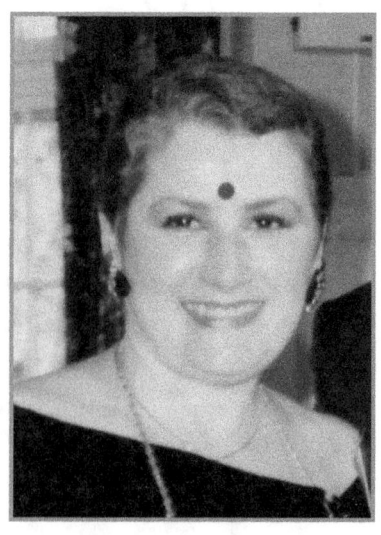

3 BONUS Reasons for Women (continued)

Your neck will finally look long enough for you to wear those dangly earrings that you love.

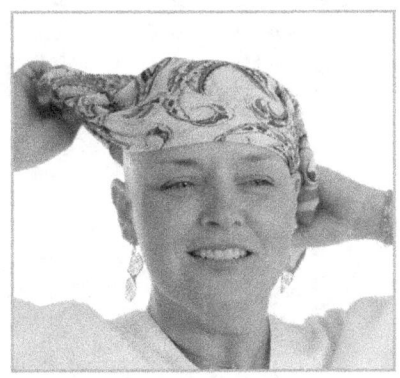

Exciting new technology enables us to clone entire locks of hair from the most minute bone fragments! Choose from our diverse collection of history's greats and future greats. Each lock has its own identifying serial number and comes with a notarized certificate of authenticity.

Available exclusively from BTU. Only $29.95 per lock. Six exciting series, plus the highly popular "Famous Couples" (priced at $59.95 for a pair of locks).

Check locks desired @ $29.95:

Eastern Greats	European Monarchs	Great Women
___ Confucius	___ Lorenzo de Medici	___ Elizabeth I
___ Gandhi	___ Louis XIV	___ Jeanne d'Arc
___ Genghis Khan	___ Pope Pius V	(Note: Tips singed)
___ Marco Polo		___ Lady Godiva
		(Supplementary fee)

	Mythical Greats	
The Great War	___ Big Foot	Future Greats (as of 1990)
___ Hitler (limited mustache locks available)	___ Godiva's Horse	___ Barbara Bush
	___ Kris Kringle	___ Bill Clinton
___ Mussolini	___ Yeti (The Abominable Snowman)	___ Mikhail Gorbachev
___ George Patton		___ Ronald Reagan

Famous Couples @ $59.95

___ Antony & Cleopatra	___ Henry VIII & Anne Boleyn
___ The Donald & Ivana	___ Napoleon & Josephine
(Remember: It was 1990!)	___ James Carville & Mary Matalin

Total Amount of Order _____

Great Hairs of History

Letter received with first (and only) order
(From my sister, who sent it to cheer me up when I was bald)

Ima Gotta Nohair
25 Glabrous Rd.
Calvous, BA 99999

Dear BTU Lady:

I'm not gunna wait another minit fer yer wonnaful offer. I'm gunna pay ya $29.95 fer all dat wonnaful hair to put on my head.

See, my Billy Bob wuz runnin aroun wit dis blond bimbo. So I sez, Ima, I sez, ya gotta be a blond. So I pours Clorox on my head, but I don't like da color. So I has dis bottle of brown dye fer dis dress. See, dis dress was blue, but my Billy Bob sees dis bimbo on TV wit a brown dress an he near goes crazy. So I sez, Ima, I sez, ya gotta have a brown dress.

So I buys dis brown dye so I kin color my dress. But I says, Ima, yer hair needs dis dye more dan yer dress. So I pours dis brown dye on my head. But my han was shakin a bit affer dat las gin, so I splashes it around a bit an it comes out kina streaky, ya know? So I says, Ima, ya gotta do sumpin fast, fore Billy Bob comes back from his buzness trip.

See Billy Bob, he hasta go on dese buzness trips all da time. When he comes back, he jus drops in his chair an wants a cuppala beers. If I wanna hop in da sack wit him I gotta intize him. So I says, Ima, ya gotta do sumpin fast about yer hair. Ya gotta get sumpin good fer yer hair.

So I ax Maria. See Maria, she knows everthin about everthin. She even went to school til she wuz 14. So Maria says, Ima, ya gotta get sumpin made jus fer hair. So I says, Ima, ya gotta go to K-Mart an get sumpin good jus fer yer hair.

So I goes to K-Mart an I buys dis stuff made jus fer hair. It wuz gonna make my hair da color of hunny. (Dis bimbo who picks up Billy Bob fer his last buzness trip, she has hair like hunny.) An ya know what dat stuff jus fer hair duz? IT MAKES ALL MY HAIR FALL OUT!

So now I ain't got no more Clorox, no more brown dye, no more hunny hair stuff, an NO MORE HAIR. Den I sees yer ad fer dis wunnaful hair an I says, Ima, ya gotta do sumpin fast fore Billy Bob comes back from his buzness trip.

Well, I sits rite down an rites ya dis chek fer $29.95 an I says, Ima, now ya gotta pick da kina hair ya want.

Well, I says, Ima, dis BTU lady she mus be pretty nice, so she probly let ya pick yer own kina hair. So now we gotta do dis order. So here it iz.

I want two hairs from dis Confuscius guy cuz Maria says he wuz smart. Den I want tree hairs from dis Gandhi guy cuz I never could sit down an cross my legs. Den I want some hairs from da Pope so I kin be blest. Den I want lotsa hair from dis Barbara Bush lady cuz Maria says den I kin talk at dis fancy girls collig. But den I wants a hole buncha hair from dat Lady Godiva so I kin intize Billy Bob. Den I wants two hairs from dis Hitler guy so if Billy Bob duznt intize I gonna zap him!

Tank ya very much.
Ima G. Nohair

May 11, 1990

Dear Ms. Nohair:

Thank you for your recent order for "The Great Hairs of History." The response to our direct mail campaign has been gratifying. (That means it makes us feel good.) It has proven that our fine-tuned targeting techniques really work. (That means we are making money on this deal.)

Based on our carefully designed research, we knew who our prime audience was and we went after them! Your order and others like it support our P.T. Barnum theory of marketing. We want you to know how much we value you as a customer (and as a source of future orders).

Speaking of which, let me congratulate you on your fine and intelligent selection from "The Great Hairs of History." It takes us additional time to process such a customized order and normally such customization would carry an additional charge.

CANCER: A Coping Guide

However, the poignancy (it brought tears to our eyes) of your letter and your plight has caused us to waive (you don't have to send more money) the additional charge and expedite (hurry up) your order. Ms. Nohair, BTU wants to put you out of your misery as quickly as possible.

The enclosed lock has hair from Barbara Bush (the white ones), from Hitler (the shorter black ones), from Confucius and Gandhi (may be difficult to pick out, as their hair was so fine they appeared bald to some folks), and of course, from Lady Godiva (the long ones).

Unfortunately, Pope Pius V is temporarily out of stock, but don't worry. I have personally arranged for my mother to make a novena on your behalf and this will bring you blessings equal to the Pope's hair.

We at BTU wish you luck with your new hair. Although we normally do not offer personal advice along with our order fulfillment (you send us money, we mail you hair) service, I feel compelled (I can't help myself) to make a suggestion to you. Tell Billy Bob if you catch him with the blonde bimbo again, you're cutting off his crown jewels. Then tell him Hitler made you say this.

Very truly yours,
Stella Baldi
Customer Service Manager, BTU

CANCER: A Coping Guide

Acknowledgments

Thank you to all my fellow cancer survivors (and sadly, some who did not survive) for sharing your stories and your feelings with me over the decades since I was diagnosed.

Special thanks to the late Lyn Goldberg who helped me face my own cancer with humor and determination. You were my role model. I hope I have lived up to your example.

Thanks also to Becky Eckstein, Lynne Fraser, Joe Petteruti and my husband, Jagdish Sachdev, for providing those extra sets of eyes to edit this book. I'm sure it wasn't as much fun as editing my social satire, but it will very likely help many people cope with a disease that will eventually touch us all.

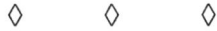

Notes

Notes

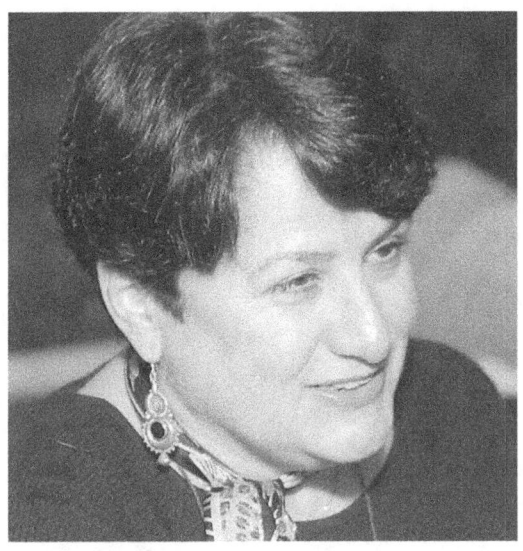

About the Author

After graduating from Brown University, Elaine M. Decker lived and worked in the metro NY area for 25 years. She was diagnosed with breast cancer in 1990, the same year as her second marriage. She kept a journal of her treatment with the intention of eventually sharing it.

A New Jersey native, Ms. Decker relocated to Providence, RI in 1992, where she lives with her husband and cats. She recently retired from nonprofit management. This followed earlier careers in marketing and communications. Retirement heralds her career as a freelance writer.

Much of her work is social satire, but she also writes on serious topics. Her writing has appeared in *The New York Times*, *Marketing News* and *The Privacy Journal*. Her previous book, *Retirement Sparks*, is comprised of selections from her blog RetirementSparks.blogspot.com. Her retirement column appears in the RI publication, *Prime Time.*